My patients raised me

This is a work of fiction. No identification with actual persons (living or deceased), places, institutions, buildings, and products is intended or should be inferred.

My patients raised me

ISBN 979-8-9895177-2-5 (softcover)
ISBN 979-8-9895177-3-2 (ebook)

I would like to dedicate this book to

The patients who entrusted in me their stories and livelihood.

The many mentors who raised me.

My parents.

Mama Nguyen and Papa Lee for raising my child, when I could not.

My wife, for everything under the moon and sun.

Tables of Contents

Preface

In medical school, every student goes through their clinical clerkships, where they are introduced to the responsibilities of each specialty. It is a humbling experience uniquely shared between physicians, allowing the student to experience the awe of what each specialty has to offer, as well as stare into the deep ravine of knowledge that one must master to become a healing physician. The journey takes one year. By the end of the year and the numerous exams, the student is usually transformed. Their clinical reasoning is expanded, their specialty goals narrowed, their wits and passion tested. How this experience changes the person is usually unpredictable.

Knowing this would be a transformative experience, I took it upon my charge to document my journey through the clinical clerkships with poetry. I allowed myself to feel passionately about my experiences, reflecting upon patient encounters and my own thoughts and insecurities. It was a privilege to be able to a part of so many patients' healing journeys, as well as their discussions and experiences with life and death.

This collection is my reflection upon these experiences. Any patient identifiers have been thoroughly scrubbed and removed, meaning this is ultimately a work of fiction. Any similarities with actual persons (living or deceased) are purely coincidentally and is not intended. This work of fiction contains no medical advice and should not be treated as any scholarly piece of work. It is not a reflection of any institution, individual, or living culture. It is simply art for the sake of art.

Humbly, I sincerely hope you are able to enjoy it as such.

PART I

an ambitious goal

Each patient has given
so much to me,
yet I could only afford
less than a minute -
a poet's recollection.

Forgive me for failing to capture it all,
for putting the finite
in infinity

Innocence

A child lays on a bed
in the hospital
surrounding by
jargon.

Words without meaning
sends more uncertainty
shooting up her spine —
she struggles to breathe.

Gripping mom's fingers
until they're blue at the tip,
the only translator
in this alien hospital room
with these nightmarish mutterings.

A mother shields a daughter's innocence
protecting her from a vocabulary assault.
The crisis in her body is enough.
The mind needs her rest.

translated

The grass begs the rabbit,
"come lie next to me.
let the weary seep from your bones
into the roots of my soil."

But the rabbit couldn't leave the shade
of her chosen barberry bush -
trade her safety and seclusion
for rest in pasture,
though free and green.

"Thank you, kind friend", she replies
her nose twitching in the sun,

"but my bones can bear the weight.
And as long as they can, so must I."

Counting Grass

I couldn't possibly count
the Blades of Grass on the lawn
and even if I managed to
new life would have sprung
and some more may have passed.

Between these living green
are so many more creatures,
smaller, smaller, then smallest
and it occurs to me that of all these lives
I could have been assembled into,

I've been gifted with me.

this body —
granted with the gift of taste, smell
sight and hearing, all of which to feel
what it means to be loved
and to love in return,

but all with it, pain.

And between the two I exist
knowing I owe the living the courtesy
of all the grace I have to offer
but also the knowledge that life is balance
and I am only able to heal so much.

...if you were to live forever...

This morning I found my walk into the hospital
littered with pill bugs,
otherwise lovingly called
the Roly Poly.

Did you also know,
its scientific name is far more sinister:
Armadillidium Vulgare?

Did you know it molts twelve selves in its lifetime?
That it spends most its life under the moon
alongside the dead and decaying,
making mulch of the mortified,
returning back to ashes all beings
within its reach?

I didn't know all that
before this morning.

I best be more careful on my morning walks in.

Those that dwell on the shore
are dependent on the waves.
That much is clear.
Dependent on it for their food,
for their transport,
their safety,
their blood.

Those on land
are gifted with
the illusion of control.
That by leaving the ocean
we have left
the waves
that come with it.

the pulse

But we were born from the ebbs and flows,
that washed us onto her shores:
forced to survive
the searing sun.
Saltless.
Our body doesn't know
how to forget —
or maybe it just doesn't wish to.

The waves are still there,
but they are within us,
beating, beating, beating.
The shore may bring with it
the carcasses of the dead.
But it is also our most powerful reminder
of where we are from.

Like Water

Medicine is not linear,
it is circular,
revising and changing
over and over —
remembering and forgetting
then finding new again.

Like water, it finds its home
temporary, over hot rocks,
boiling into mist,
giving life along the riverbed,
while assaulting the salty shore.

And through it all
I am grateful to have drank
from her source.

I await to see
how it will change me.
I await to see
what parts of her I keep
and what parts of her
I must return.

My student clinician oath

I will be true to myself.
And in the thickest thicket,
I will remain the bravest cricket.

Early mornings

I wake before the roosters
and the roasters, too, for that matter.

I wake before my body does,
before the moon has had her fill of night.

Before the sun and her winged chariot
evaporates the carpet of dew.

I don't wake because I have to.
I wake because I mean to.

In the newborn nursery

I am grateful to have been a parent
before holding onto these newborns.
The trials of fatherhood have taught me
more than any instruction ever could.

How to hold them,
swaddle them,
sing to them.
Listen.

How to center myself,
to project confidence and love
through the glove and the gown.

I think it makes a difference
knowing your arms are their world.

my patients raised me

She spoke quietly to an audience
in stochastic whispers.
She said "my children raised me
the way they needed me"

Her "wisdom" was bidirectional,
unique to their collective weaknesses.
They know.

Though most of it
hardly matters now,
especially since she'll go soon.
"Any day now," she says.

The only lessons worth holding
are the ones
that will keep them strong.

Forgive the many mistranslations
along the way.
But maybe one day
they'll find meaning in the blunders.

Maybe one day
they'll have children of their own
and they will be raised by them, too.

all we take

they calculate that over one lifetime,
we take a staggering 600 million breaths,
that's 300 million liters of air
to fuel 3 billion heartbeats.

and yet it all feels so short
by the end.
or at least so I've heard.

the great metronome
continues to click
as I live my life,
almost blissfully unaware.

	We all start somewhere,
amateur	as *amateurs* do.
	But why is that word
	so synonymous with mediocre,
	when it was originally born of love?
amatore	*amatore*,
amare	*amare*,
	"one who loves" en Français.
	We all start somewhere.
	But more importantly,
	we all get to where we want to be
	through trials of love.

One   for   one

Undoubtedly,
there is simply not enough space
in my little noggin
to store all the knowledge
medicine has to offer.

So naturally,
some space must be made —
sacrifices if you will.

I'll happily trade the memories
of my kindergarten days,
of my high school classmate's name,
the license plate of my first car,
the facial details of my first love.

Those are the easy swaps
For potentially lifesaving knowledge.

The harder ones
are the ones that have not yet been born
or the ones born
without my presence:

discounted lunches at IKEA with my toddler

his tiny fingers sifting through warmed sand

a beaming smile on a sunny day at the park…

27

Those memories
are the ones I wish to hold onto.

But some knowledge is deadly enough
it must be prioritized,

bearing great cost to man
and to me.

Story I

When does a story begin?

Is it when we are born?
But surely before then, too.

A mother recounts her desire for you,
your journey to the womb,
the wanting and effort that
guaranteed your existence.

How far back then, do we go?

PART II

dying

The act of dying
is a subtle
magic trick
because it is always
one step behind
living.
Looming in the shadows
of our most precious memories;
we fear not
what comes next,
but rather leaving all
that we have built
behind.

Linguistic decisions

Here, in English,
we are taught to *make*
a decision.

"Put your nickel down,"
I am often told in the clinic.

Fitting for the land of innovation,
the pioneers of medicine,
to focus on shaping destiny.

But it provides me solace
that elsewhere, in Spanish, they say

> *toma* una decisión
> (*take* a decision),

knowing full well
there are different paths;
and that taking one
may often preclude the other.

A finality that is lost
in the English translation…

Perhaps my favorite though,
is how it is said in German

    that a decision is *met.*

That resonates with me the most:
the concept of meeting a decision
invokes two parties,
whether the party
is the physician and the patient
or the person and a higher being.

That somehow decisions
are intertwined with fate.

That you are never alone
when choosing.

Consequences

Both face a path
beyond scientific surety.

One is bleeding from his bladder,
but an artery in his heart,
is blocked, too.
We can't stop the bleed,
for his heart is too weak.
And we can't operate on the heart
for he'd need meds that risk
a 3-month-long bleed.
So he sits and waits
for a heart attack that is surely
to come.
A consequence to force someone's hand.

The other has a clot
right next to his right collar bone
with a straight path to his lungs.
It would stop his breath,
it might even stop his heart.
But we cannot catch it
because his liver has failed him,
so he is unable to clot.
He finds himself having to decide
whether to bleed
or risk
not being able
to breathe.

35

Air

Some days
air
is all you have
and often
those days
air
is all
you need.

Turning over

I left home at 18,
each of my cells
still brimming with evidence
of my heritage:

my stomach filled with my father's cooking,
my lungs saturated with the scent of New York,
my bones built from her dairy farms,
my hair wet from her week-long rains.

I walked differently;
my thoughts were, too.
I talked differently
than I ought to.

But now that I am older
so little of my home
is left in me.

My colon was the first to go -
turned over in 3 days,
wasted in the sewage system of Missouri.

My skin didn't last long either -
about two months later,
enough pieces to replace me
were strewn on loose clothing,
or scrubbed away with body wash…

My lungs adapted well to the new climate,
and by the time I returned to New York,
they could not recognize it as home.

If you dug into my bones,
you might've found some home in me
even ten years after I'd left.
But now even that
would be a treasure amongst
the trabeculae.

I am living in a new shell.
My brain knows where I am from,
but cannot find any evidence
elsewhere in my body.
It replays memories
of me, laying on my front porch,
but it cannot place my hands -
younger, unwrinkled.

The finger that traced the clouds back then
is replaced by the one I own now.

Question from a 99-year-old woman

You ask me
if taking a wrong pill
every now and then is bad for you.

Well, you tell me.

You're the one
who has made it to ninety-nine.
I'm the one
with all the learning to do.

Ringing

I forget to close the car door.
And my car reminds me —
interrupts my routine as I grab my scrubs
and prepare to head home for the night.

I close it —
find myself gifted with silence yet again,
composed, but for you.

Far away, the beeping never stops for you.

Starting from the inside of your car, then
the ambulance's sirens and
the radios hanging on hips;
a nurse yells 'vitals'
as you rush into the ER.
And every room you would see thereafter.

Beeping

either yours or another's,

Incessant

until you can't even complete a thought
when that is all you want to do.
As you stare at the curtain,
their muted colors so lifeless
your gaze fintds itself
the only human thing in the room…

When I am to pass.
Let me pass gently,
let me slip away
without the sound of machines.

with a smile
and warm blankets.
A man can dream.

But if all else fails,
and nothing is and no one comes
just please
for the love of God,
before unplugging the machine.
Turn off the damn alarms.

Walls

The walls vibrate from the echoed screams,
the ceaseless monitors,
the shouted orders that are launched
within them.

But how much can the walls hold?
They're only so thick.
Where does the rest of the sound travel?
Does it stay tethered on my scrubs?
Or does some of it seep into my skin?

Do I end up carrying some of it home?

wandering in the mind

The Colorado forests have taught me
the valuable lesson of how easy it is
to be lost in the woods.

How if one wants to remember a path
sure and true,
they must either create a diligent map
or carve straight through.

Memories are much the same.
For the only sure way to recall facts quickly
would be to tear down the forest entirely.
Replace it with roads and
cars and
infrastructure, all
designed for efficiency,
trading chaos for speed.

An unpruned mind may be a beautiful thing,
but it has no place
in this hospital setting.

lessons of the hand

There are hidden clues in medicine.
And some believe they reside in the hand.

"Clubbing" of the fingers,
predicts an issue with the lungs.
Darkened spots on the fingertips,
a potential infection hidden in the heart.
A darkened stripe on the nail
a potential skin cancer.

One individual I worked with
would pay particular attention to the hand,
looking for skin tenting
as signs of dehydration,
a resting tremor
concerning for Parkinson's,
redness of the palms
as a sign of liver failure.

He would stress the importance
of a handshake with the patient
beyond the formal expectations.

"Did you know the sailors
used to check for syphilis
with a single handshake,"
enlarged lymph nodes are a later sign
of infection…

I've also come to also appreciate
you learn, too, about who they are
beyond their medical needs:

the presence of callouses
with hard, manual labor;

colorful playful nails
with a sense of decorum;

a strong firm handshake,
a father who stressed it so.

Handshake

I shook hands with a man who was about to enter
the world again, his world again

full of its fears,
away from the care
of our hands
and watchful eyes.

Here, the walls have alarms,
there are medicines
to keep the shakes away.

Out there, he says he only has
his own devices,
and he's afraid
they may not be enough.

the placebo effect

The moon is 1,079 miles wide,

a quarter the size of the earth.

I know this.

And yet tonight it lays larger and brighter on the horizon

than I have ever known it to.

Brighter than it ought to be.

Bigger than it is.

To hell with the man who tells me

how the moon ought to look tonight —

that it's just the trick of the light.

Who are they to say

how the moon looks to me?

Who are they to know

how it makes me feel?

The Cosmic Dawn

They say the faint whispers beyond our planet:
vibrating planets, clashing meteors
millions of miles away
arrive all at once, in what they refer to as
the cosmic dawn.

But only if one has the patience to listen.
Only if we embrace and surround ourselves
with silence.

There is a cosmic dawn in every patient I see
and my biggest charge is to hold myself
and listen.

Et. Al.

is inscribed on my stethoscope.
As it is placed on your chest,
its thick black cord reverberating,
I am reminded of the voices
that stood up for me,
the hands that reached out for mine,
the shoulders of giants.

And importantly, too,
the many of yours,
some waiting just outside the door
to hear the verdict,
and the others that plan to visit later
when the doctors are done doctoring.

Even those who have passed,
whose memories you carry with you
to guide you through these trying times.

Two villages meet
at the diaphragm
of the stethoscope.
A heart always beats
for more than just one.

Jaundice

The morning sun's rays
have overstayed their welcome,
made your glowing skin
their new home,
mistaking it,
staining it,
with its loving light —
clinging,
unwilling
to let go.

Your eyes were so yellow…

The mourn

I have found the amber grain
the light beyond the veil.
It is not the kind of light one sees
it's the kind of light one feels.

Can you promise me you'll keep it safe –
use its rays to grow that within you?
Though on second thought
it is too delicate and too heavy
for someone only accustomed
to the morning sun.

The night before the storm

He can hear the horsemen's hooves
preceded by a red glazing the sky.
As if the darkness has weight,
he feels a gravity
pulling.

He is kneeled against mortality
and his balled-up fists gripping tight
foreshadowing
a rigidness he knows
is waiting for him.

He wishes he could stand up now.
Not to call for help;
he is more ready than he expected.
But to comb his hair and tie his shoes
so he can walk into that black hole

Proudly
and head on.

Silence

Day breaks
and morning comes.
Rays of sunshine
piercing through hospital panes,
sharp, and unslowed by floating dust,
they settle on mottled grey hands -
colder than the blanket that now covers them;
the coldest ones in the room.

Silence, for the Queen, at last.
A life was lost today.
As mourning is unveiled as uproar -
restless nights await the family.
Dust, unsettled.
A choir of wailing.
Songs will be sung.

The sky bled last night,
lacerated clouds allowing heaven's colors
to seep through the lenses.
And we find we're fortunate enough
to watch your soul pass.
I hope as you leave our finite world
you are graced with infinite peace

Story II

When is a story worth being told?
Our lives are filled
with so many adventures
our minds remember those it deems worthy to.
But how does it so choose
which stories are worth being told?
And why does it hold onto what it does?
And what holds us back from saying them aloud?

It's true that some say
recording these events
somehow brings more meaning
to the lived experiences,
to my lived experience.

It's also a universal fact
that they say matter cannot be created.

It's a pity they give so little guidance
on whether any of this matters –
if there is any meaning to matter, itself.

That is what I truly want to know.

PART III

the language of the dead

Death is deaf to
the pleas of loved ones,
whose vocal cords
cannot yet pierce
our thick skin.

It is blind
to all the caring souls outside
struggling so hard
to push life in
through the lungs
through the blood.

It is not uncaring,
it is simply naïve
to what we hold dear.
The body knows only molecules.
It speaks only the language it knows.

my first autopsy

I learned you drank every day,
as evidenced by your clean
aorta — free of plaques.

I know you had a vasectomy,
as evidenced by the post-procedure marks
in your testicles.

I know your urinary habits
likely meant shorter walks in the park.
I know this, because of long-standing
prostate growths.

But ultimately, I know
you died
from the growing mass
in your brain.

Evidenced by the large surgical scars on your scalp,
some healed,
some less so;
the staples holding your skull plates together;
the missing segment of your cranium…

I never knew you in life.
But in death, I am intimately aware
of every lesion you had on your body
and inside of it.

It is strange for me
to hold this knowledge
when so few have held it before.
And in some guilty way,
it does not feel like I should hold it
if I can do no harm,
but also do no good.

Necklace

Mortality is having a necklace
placed on your neck as a child
when your head was still small
but your soul a bolder you.
It hung loosely then,
when you were a pirate on the playground
dying over and over again in the vast seas.
Fearless. Immortal.
When you skied down the slopes
straight as lightning.

But with age, the line becomes taut
and the chain rubs against your thickening skin
until one day you realize
you cannot take it off.
A new hesitancy grips you:
transforming vastness to roughness;
lightning makes your heart skip a beat.

Each day forth you have a choice:
to fear the day the necklace gets too tight
constricting your precious air
or to wear it proudly,
as your ancestors did,
a gift from your parents
to experience all that is beautiful and transient.
An insignia of infinity

Built

We are built different
and we are built broken

Dinner

Coming home
to a warm dinner
after dissecting a brain
or slicing into
fixed breast tissue
is a strange sort of thing.

It is a kind of feeling
so few are privy to.
It is the kind of grime
I find I cannot wash away.

I will admit
the knowledge I gained
was fair trade.

At the cost
of some evening joy,
I have the opportunity
so few have.

I have an opportunity
to do real good.

I am not ready for the silence

I wanted you.
Before you were born,
you were wanted. You
were already loved.

And as your little fingers grew,
ultrasound after ultrasound, I
find the weights disparate.
I cannot believe
how much of me you hold
in that tiny corporealness.
I need you.

My life, forever altered
by your mere existence.
My world, infinitesimally smaller —
keenly aware you'll soon outgrow
these thickened walls.

You already try to pull away.

I am not ready.

where does the cold go?

At twenty something weeks,
you passed away.

A congenital heart defect
meant you would not make it
to your birth date.

Rather, you find yourself
on a pathologist's bench,
pulseless
breathless
cold —
so cold in fact
it appears you are shaking.
But I know that cannot be.
It's just the vibration of the fan
humming above the table.

My liveliness suddenly feels jarring
next to what little of life you were given.
So, my gloved hands cover your backside,
in a way a father's would.
But the warmth is only drained from me
without anywhere else to go.

There is no amount of warmth
enough to satisfy the dead.

That which stays

As the observations are made,
a diagnosis is reached.
And you were lowered back into
the formalin you arrived in.
But enough of you remains.

It is not something
a normal man is meant to carry.
Nor is it something
someone who aspires to be exceptional
expects to.

It is an experience that once had,
requires safeguarding
in the safest quadrants of human nature,
the quietest silos of remembrance,
next to the marbles reminiscent of childhood,
next to the recipes passed on from grandma.

Facts

It takes time to appreciate scientific writing. It first reads so dull, objective to a fault, littered with math and ever-specifying jargon, as if humanity was stripped from its prose. One wonders whether the reader was ever considered since its contents lack so much as gentleness — its words lack song.

But these attributes are precisely
what I have come to love.
The flowering tree is only a grandeur
because the barked trunk lifts it so.

To utter statements so proudly as facts
requires more than belief,
it requires knowledge, paid and tested.
To usher a theory requires layers
of statements on statements
ideas not born iron-clad, but iron-proved.
A published paper wishes to be unperishable.
As truth stands and stands,
still.

Unlucky

I suppose it is hard to reckon with
the how and the why
some cancers can arise to be so deadly
while others are left so benign.

The how is what keeps the scientists up at night;
what fuels their lofty goals of savior.
But the why keeps restless the patient.
The why is whispered in prayer.

And though our scientific endeavor
may someday discover
the how
I feel we may never uncover enough
to explain away the
the why.

Aren't there any other options?

I'm sorry.
Science doesn't work that way
and if you spend long enough with her
you wonder if she even works at all
in the face of such complexity.

It feels
like trying to understand
the ocean
One spoonful
at a time.

Wishes of the many

Death is not a democracy
the failure of a few cells
is   often   just   enough.
The   body   is   frail.

Cumulative consequence

It unlikely the painful lesion that kills you
nor the largest malformation make your final straw.
We are designed to notice the large,
and adapted to tackle the acute.

It is the slow and insidious,
the poison confused with living
that tricks the body so thoroughly,
it incorporates it as its own.

It is the cumulative consequence
of what we consider ours
that takes its final toll.

Tell-tale signs of the sword

Those that wield the sword
carry with them callouses,
scars of the sort,
battle-stories,
a steel nerve.

Just as those who wield the scalpel
find their necks ache,
their backs just a little too tight,
perhaps a curt tongue.

But there is a weight they carry
one that requires
some compassion to recognize.

Holding one's life
at the flick of a wrist
is no easy task.
There are some matters that require
the sword,
but we often forget
the hands and the minds
that wield it.

What fills the bowels?

I wonder what your bowels hold,
aside from the sutures placed in them.
Can the thousands of nerves residing there
hold a memory?
Can they remember what the outside air felt like?
The warm glow of the surgical light?
The vibrating sounds of surgeons?
Or does it awaken afraid each day
of the numerous holes in its mucosa,
terrified and confused of the foreign stitches
a most unnatural intrusion?

The drive home

On my way home I see
the clouds have caught
the last few rays of the setting sun —
the short-lived red tips
dress the blue,
while beads of geese navigate
the skyline.

How comforting it is to know
we all yearn for home.

A crescent moon finds her way to the forefront;
the horizon fades to a darker hue.

The low laying mountains belong somewhere else,
perhaps to Santa Fe.

There is a memory there.

Story III

When does a story end?
You are you when you fall asleep
not because of the promise of awakening
but because you are
you even when you're unconscious.

You are you even before you can remember,
and even after you forget.
And if you hold memories of you
under the influence,
doesn't that mean you were you when you
stumbled your way home?

The you in this hospital bed –
your son is saying is not you;
your wife says she cannot recognize it.

But your tears say different.
You are you even though you are not
the same.

Who is to say
when I am not me,
anymore?

PART IV

healing

After a cut
the skin seems
to remember
how to
grow back.
As long as not
too much
was taken away.
As long as there's still
something left
to hold onto.
And as long as
enough time was spent
nurturing it.

Body part I

the nerves inside me
do not see
the rising and setting
of the sun.
they do not know
when to wake,
or
more importantly
when to rest.
it is up to me
to remind them
by eating right
resting right
moving right…

Body part II

..And I listened to my body
but I couldn't hear a thing.

to which my body replied,
"we've shared a home together…
and yet you know
so little of me"

After the accident

Your left arm is still stiff
after the accident.
The physical reminder of all you've lost
in the blink of your eyes:

Your daughter.

     Your appetite.

         Your normalcy.

As if the devil reached for each of you in the car,
and somehow only you
managed to rip free of his grip,
though not all of you
was so lucky.
A mark of his touch remains,
a tethered reminder of an unspeakable place.

The arm makes living so very challenging.
Not just because of the pain,
but because the memories —
they should be living, too.

The memories of living, two.

Between

Some acts of kindness
lie in between
only I am able to,
and I am only able to

as you approach unremarkable

Many of your labs
continue to improve,
approaching what we term
'unremarkable.'

So it is, in the hospital,
as doctors strive to be exceptional
the patient strives to be
'unremarkable.'

Your mustache, though
will forever remain
absolutely
remarkable.

I don't mean to make this about me
but there is so little left of living
after leaving the hospital.

It is like I have left more there
than I ever imagined I could give.

All the decisions I had in me
are used up.
The fatigue and wear
start to tear at the seams
and all I wish is to unravel
upon a comfy couch.

Left of living

With each leaving I find
more and more and more of me left
on the bed
between my wife
and my child's little toes.

My imprint stays impressed
upon the sheets
just a little while longer —
the magics of longing.

And I find myself thinking
of how their mornings look
when mine are so far away.
There is much of my life I enjoy,
but   the   leaving.

Dreams of a moth

In the mornings I awake
I can barely discern when the black
of my coffee reaches the tip
of my mug.
The time of day so many sleep through
I confuse with morning.
The warmth of the day that graces me
comes from this dark liquid,
a poor substitute for the sun.

To refer to medicine as a calling
is to glorify the streetlight to a moth.
I'm sure the fluorescent lights call to it too.
I'm sure it believes
the moon is there to grace it
with its bountiful glory.

That is not to say the act of medicine
is not meaningful.
But in context,
it remains to be seen
any
more
meaningful.

"I'll grow ugly one day," she said
"Perhaps," said the man staring back
"But not in my eyes"

Entropy: a gradual decline to disorder

Those in medicine defy entropy
all the time.
We were bred to build
cathedrals of knowledge
to perform miracles against nature
such that a new
entropic state of survival
is attained.

So it is not surprising
we find it so difficult
to sit in this disordered state –
to stop building
and instead,
just be.

Staring upwards at the stars
clear as the night sky could be,
I am reminded that tomorrow will soon come
and a thought so frightening finds me:

Do I have what it takes to weather it?

Not the storm, nor the wind –
those I have spent
my entire life preparing for
failure followed by fibrosis, meant
to cure my skin as thick as hide...

No, rather the sun rays breaking past
blue skies, cloudless,
direct sun onto my aging skin
reminding my cells
I have a chance to enjoy life
and be happy…

Would I know what to do then
and do I have the courage to feel the warmth,
expose myself to garish amber rays
and not retreat into a hospital?
A courage I was born with
but time has allowed me to forget.

My path here has ill prepared me
for a stilled mind that watches the day pass
only to transform to night,
a beautiful meaninglessness
before the sun eventually rises.

we were raised

In medicine, we're taught to build-
place each plank on top of another.
And these mental acrobatics
may one day have us thinking
we were born this way —
like acclimated children at the top of a stairwell
except fluent in a language dead and foreign to most.

But we were acorns once,
and we need not forget
that underneath the carpeted floors,
covered in blood and wine,
are rough and bare oak panels
and the nails used to raise them

G   r   i   e   f

We find can describe grief that way,
like having a reliable toolset
but misplacing the screwdriver.
A car that still runs,
but doesn't climb the hill the same.

A new reality sets in
the new "whole"
just doesn't feel such.

Like a lobster shrinking inside his shell,
alien, unwelcomed space appears.

Were there a word for it,
it would be grief.

Desperate

Like a miner along the Colorado river,
I am desperately trying to hold onto
as many experiences as I can
to learn as much as my patients
are willing to teach me.
Knowing full well
I can only remember so much,
that a bucket is meant to release water just as much
as it is meant to hold onto it.
And letting go is often the hardest part

32-year-old male

It is not lost upon me
that   each   day
I   inch   closer
to   becoming
the   patient.

Habit

When we pass
People tend to remember
that which is habit of ours
and that which takes so little
effort.
May I be fortunate enough
that my being kind
and loving
will be remembered so

Story IV

Time seems a cruel thing.
It takes that which was so important
and turns it
into fibrosis,
into lysis,
into dust.

Our tepid memories attempt to take
what was there,
but it's too dependent
on blood and body,
so they fade, too.

Books and pictures so rarely carry with them
anything more than two-dimensionality,
and fewer and fewer people
stay long enough
to extract anything else.

It is almost as if Time
begs us to forget.
As if she is teaching us
over and over again
that each moment is not beautiful
because it can be remembered,
but because
it must be experienced.